THE HIGH PERFORMANCE MALE

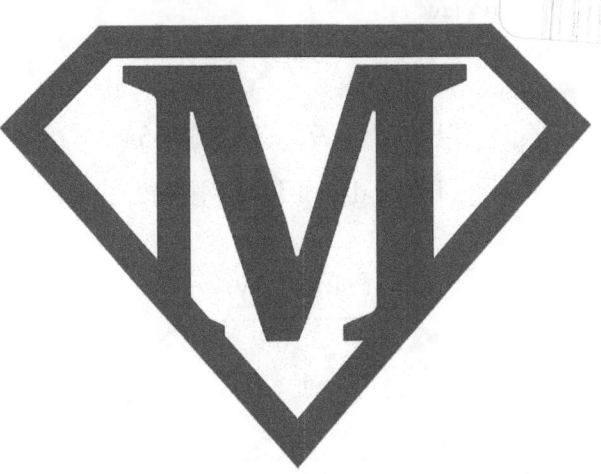

High-octane strategies to accelerate performance…
in and out of the bedroom…
for men over 40

DESMOND EBANKS, MD

THE HIGH PERFORMANCE MALE

High-octane strategies to accelerate performance...
in and out of the bedroom...for men over 40

Copyright © 2017 Desmond Ebanks

ISBN-13: 978-1548614454

ISBN-10: 1548614454

Printed by:

The Five Star Group, LLC
10403 Coachouse Place • Louisville, KY 40223
www.TheFiveStarGroup.com

For more information on The Five Star Group, including finding out how you can publish your own book, visit TheFiveStarGroup.com or call (800) 645-8642.

Dedication

This book is dedicated to the memory of my parents, Walter and Melonee Ebanks, whose generous spirits would want it shared with everyone who wants to experience extraordinary performance and the power of well-being.

Here's What's Inside...

Acknowledgements

I would like to express my deepest gratitude to the many people with whom I have worked and learned from to produce the ideas, concepts and strategies that are presented in this book.

To my lovely wife and best friend, Cynthia, none of this would be possible without you.

To my beautiful daughter, Neena, for whom my love knows no bounds.

To my clients and patients, you put your trust in me to assist you throughout the last 30 years. You have been my source of inspiration and I have learned from you how to work towards perfecting my craft.

Chapter 1
The High Performance Male

As a medical doctor for over three decades, and a Board Certified specialist in internal medicine, I have had the good fortune to have made an impact in the lives of many people. Ranging from the life-saving events in the emergency room to helping maintain a viable workforce in occupational medicine, to helping people maintain their quality of life, my career has been quite rewarding.

Other than my emergency room experience, which, despite its rewards, was a very stressful way to practice medicine, I never felt like I was really in a position to "fix" anything. As an internal medicine physician, I felt like I just helped people tread water until they slowly got tired and drowned.

In conventional medicine, you're considered well if you don't have a diagnosis. The fact is many people don't have a diagnosis, but they don't feel well either. The response is typically, "Well, you're getting old, what do you expect? You're going to be tired. You're not going to be able to perform like you used to." Instead of looking for the underlying cause of why the person isn't feeling well, the conventional medicine approach is to begin prescribing medications to address the symptoms. If you're feeling a little down, an antidepressant is prescribed. Feeling a little anxious? Here's something for anxiety.

Experiencing some erectile dysfunction? Here's a prescription for some Viagra. And so on and so on.

The symptom-oriented approach of conventional medicine was becoming less and less gratifying to me. So I began searching for something different - a style of medicine that focused on getting to the root cause of the problem rather than just trying to mask the symptoms. That ultimately led me to the creation of Alternity Healthcare in 2007 to focus on a new paradigm of managing the aging process and addressing the root cause of dysfunction and disease rather than just the symptoms of them.

The evidence has been with us for decades that somewhere north of 80% of all chronic diseases, including cancers, are preventable with lifestyle modification. As a patient, if you understand lifestyle management as being the correct way to eat, the correct way to be physically active, making sure you're getting the appropriate amount of sleep, managing your stress and your hormones, you're now managing your aging process and, in the process, extending your vitality.

Moving far beyond mere wellness, I have been able to help people truly get better, not just feel better. By helping people maximize their life experience, this innovative approach addresses the natural process of aging by maintaining and extending the vitality of youth during the time of life where we typically start to see a steady, steep decline after age 40 or 50. But my story doesn't end there.

Looking at the data from all of the people I was helping to elevate their health and restore their vitality, it became increasingly clear that diminishing performance, in one aspect or another, was the real underlying problem. With the advances in the field of genomic analysis, the next logical progression in my professional journey was to utilize the information available in your DNA blueprint to specifically address performance impairing issues with targeted treatments and customized programing that can alter genetic expression. This new concept incorporates the latest genomic and epigenomic science to see your individual genetic strengths and weakness, and the influence of specific environmental triggers that can affect your results. This comprehensive approach to boosting performance and optimizing health creates sustainable solutions for long term results.

I have had the privilege to help thousands of men improve the quality of their lives. Using a combination of in depth assessment of key health parameters, realistic individualized goals, and consistent follow through, my patients have enjoyed greater virility, increased vigor, and a greater level of potency. I believe my mission is to radically improve the human condition; that is, transform average human potential into exceptional performance. This is the future of healthcare… here, now…for you.

After reading this book, my hope is that you find it helpful in answering some of your questions regarding your particular health. In the meantime, all good health to you and I do hope our paths cross soon. Enjoy the book.

Chapter 2
High Performance as a Lifestyle

What does "high performance" mean to you? To some it is dominating athletic feats, prodigious work output or energetic sexual exploits. Others might think of high-end sports cars, other types of precision machinery or luxury items. Some clothing manufacturers even refer to their fabrics as high performance for their ability to keep you cool in the heat, warm in the cold or not wrinkle when traveling. High performance can be all of those things. But, more importantly, as we will explore in this book, enhancing performance is the best method for optimizing your personal health and wellbeing, achieving your personal goals and living your life as the best version of yourself.

Your health, vitality and longevity are all directly related to the performance of every organ system in your body and, by extension, every cell in your body. Who doesn't want their heart to perform at a high level? Brain? Immune system? Gut? Lungs? Kidneys? Muscles and joints? Every part of you can be optimized. By using advanced technologies to look deeper at physiological measures down to the cellular level, disease promoting and performance sapping abnormalities can be uncovered and addressed.

Over the years I have seen thousands of men from around the world, many of them previous high performers, come to me with complaints of fatigue, depression, low sex drive, diminished work performance, accumulating body fat, reduced ability to recover after exercise, flagging mental clarity, muscle and joint pain, and feeling less healthy than five years before. Tapping into the unrealized potential within each of them, these men became aware that change was possible and that they now had a customized roadmap to the actions they needed to undertake in order to restore and rejuvenate their power as men. They came in as patients with symptoms, but were transformed into successful clients; looking better, feeling better and performing better.

By reading this book, you are invited to join a select group of individuals seeking to transform their health and lives, and are unwilling to accept mediocrity or conventional thinking with regard to their health and wellbeing. If you follow the strategies outlined in this book you will radiate confidence in your ability to handle life's challenges, melt away body fat and regain muscle mass, experience firmer erections and heightened sexual pleasure, boost your memory and brain power, and experience lifelong vitality.

Chapter 3
What Do Men Really Need?

M ore than fifty years ago the psychologist Abraham Maslow had a revolutionary impact on the field of psychology when he wrote about the Hierarchy of Needs. His theory is often portrayed as a pyramid with the most basic fundamental needs in the broad base and the concept of self-actualization at the top.

Figure 1

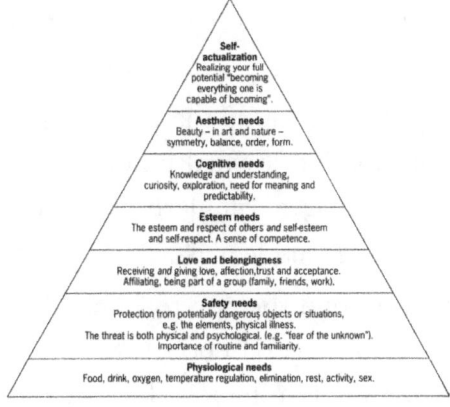

According to Maslow the four most fundamental needs include physiological needs, safety, love & friendship and self-esteem (figure 1). Critics of his theory have taken issue with Maslow's rankings; believing he may have overlooked the most essential human need; to "feel alive". Perhaps nothing makes you feel more alive than feeling younger, healthier and more vital. And nothing does all of that better for men than testosterone.

Testosterone is the primary male sex hormone, or androgen. Circulating levels of testosterone increase at the time of puberty and peak in early adulthood for men. Testosterone is responsible for men looking like men and feeling like men.

Following that peak is a gradual but steady decline in testosterone levels beginning in the mid-30's. Declining testosterone levels cause a variety of symptoms including loss of muscle mass and strength, increased belly fat, impaired brain function, disrupted sleep, loss of libido, impaired sexual function and general fatigue.

Because the loss of testosterone is gradual, these symptoms typically occur little by little, and the impact on a man's life may not be felt until his 40's, 50's or later. This is sometimes referred to as andropause, or the male menopause. This gradual decline in vitality, function and quality of life is too often attributed to "just getting old" when in reality, many of those symptoms can be reversed with proper treatment.

It is readily apparent to most that testosterone plays a crucial role in male sexual function. Sexual potency peaks along with the raging hormones of a teenager. Similarly, testosterone is essential for building and maintaining muscle mass, youthful energy and strength.

Considering testosterone therapy to improve the way you look, feel and perform would be good enough for many. In fact, testosterone therapy has resulted in improved libido and erectile function in middle-aged men. However, recent scientific evidence has demonstrated significant adverse health implications for men with low and declining testosterone levels. Numerous studies have now established a strong association between low testosterone and depression, metabolic syndrome, type-2 diabetes, osteoporosis and cardiovascular disease. In one study men with low testosterone had a nearly 50% increase in mortality over a seven year period. An unmistakable link has also been established between erectile dysfunction and the development of cardiovascular disease.

Several studies have shown that restoring testosterone to more youthful levels in middle-aged men improved insulin-sensitivity, reduced serum cholesterol, fat mass, waist circumference and inflammatory bio-markers associated with heart disease, diabetes, and metabolic syndrome. One study concluded "that testosterone treatment in men has potentially beneficial effects on virtually all of the coronary risk factors, as well as an independent anti-plaque forming action." In men with heart failure, testosterone therapy also improved functional capacity, or the ability to perform physical activity without constraint.

So why aren't more men getting testosterone therapy? Many physicians do not recognize the symptoms of low testosterone as a treatable condition. Traditionally, physicians have been reluctant to prescribe testosterone therapy in large part out of a misguided fear of increasing prostate cancer risk.

Recent evidence has called that conventional paradigm into question. A large meta-analysis out of Harvard University, as well as a collaborative review of 18 prospective studies concluded that no significant association existed between higher testosterone levels and prostate cancer risk. Conversely, studies have shown an increased risk of prostate cancer and aggressive prostate cancer in men with low testosterone levels. In a group of middle-aged men treated with testosterone and followed for more than 5 years, there was no increase in the incidence of prostate cancer and PSA levels remained stable.

In addition to the fear that prescribing testosterone would increase the risk of developing prostate cancer, physicians were also warned about increasing the risk of heart disease.

In 2014 two articles were published suggesting an increased cardiovascular risk associated with testosterone therapy. There was tremendous media hype surrounding those articles, which ultimately resulted in a warning from the FDA; a warning that was premature in my opinion.

Looking at the same data, the European Medicines Agency concluded that there was "no consistent evidence" of increased cardiovascular risks. Other research has even indicated a protective effect of testosterone on the heart.

That protective effect was reaffirmed in a large-scale study from the Veterans Affairs system, which was published in the European Heart Journal. The results suggested that treated men that reached normal levels of testosterone were 56% less likely to die, 24% less likely to have a heart attack, and 36% less likely to have a stroke than the untreated men.

In a 2017 study published in the Journal of Sexual Medicine, the authors concluded that, "Overall, we confirmed the broad and sustained benefits of testosterone replacement therapy across major quality of life dimensions, including sexual, somatic, and psychological health, which were sustained over 36 months in our treatment cohort."

Another 2017 study published in the Journal of Cardiovascular Pharmacology and Therapeutics showed a dramatic reduction in mortality, heart attack and stroke in men treated with testosterone (figure 2).

Although these studies support the safety and benefits of testosterone therapy in men, it does not mean that everyone feeling run down with low sex drive is a suitable candidate for treatment. Any man over 40 or 50 that feels off his game, run down or is experiencing any of the symptoms of low testosterone should have a thorough evaluation looking for cardiovascular disease, pre-diabetes, and osteoporosis among others. Treatment should only be prescribed by a physician experienced with testosterone therapy and the necessary monitoring of levels once therapy has begun.

Rather than narrowly focusing on just your hormone levels, a comprehensive program that includes lifestyle changes related to nutrition and exercise will expose your total health picture and help you move toward achieving optimal health.

Figure 2

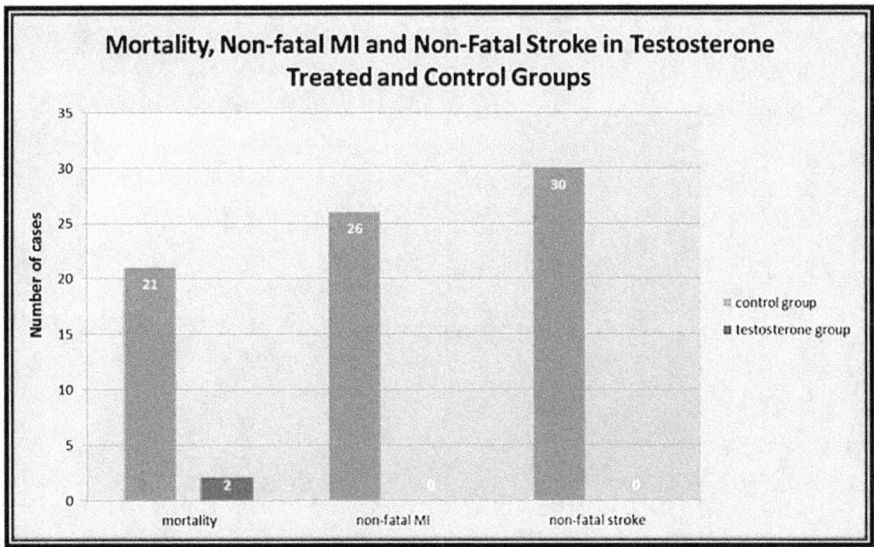

Chapter 4
Hormone Balance and Your Health

Attaining and maintaining a high performance lifestyle requires a deep understanding of the cellular mechanisms and underlying factors that can impact your performance. I have spent many years gaining this insight that, frankly, many other doctors simply don't have. One of the key strategies involves getting your hormones in balance. These hormones, when out of balance, can have serious consequences on your life. These effects include excess fat storage, interference with your ability to combat stress and focus, increased risk of diabetes and other metabolic diseases, not to mention wreaking havoc on sleep and sex life.

The body system responsible for controlling your hormones is the endocrine system. In the brain, the hypothalamus and pituitary glands act as the control centers for sending and receiving messages from your pancreas, adrenal glands, thyroid, and testicles.

Although a number of hormones can affect your physical and mental health, three of the most important ones for men to be aware of are testosterone, growth hormone, and estrogen.

Testosterone

As mentioned in the previous chapter, testosterone is a vital part of being a healthy, virile man at any age. It's what makes you strong, smart, quick and aggressive. It's what makes you a potent and virile lover. It's what gives you the drive to succeed in school, sports and business. This chapter will explore testosterone and other key hormones in greater detail.

Testosterone is what makes you feel invincible in your teens and twenties. And the decrease of testosterone in your body is what makes you feel weaker, slower and more fragile as you age. The real question is: do we have to accept declining testosterone levels, and the declining health and capability that causes, as we grow older?

Testosterone is produced in the testicles and adrenal glands and released into the blood stream. The amount of testosterone varies during the day, with the peak in the morning and the lowest production in the evening. Most of the testosterone in the circulation is tightly bound to proteins called sex-hormone binding globulin (SHBG)– only approximately 2% is available for the body's use. This portion is called the "free" testosterone. A larger portion called "bioavailable" testosterone is loosely bound to other proteins like albumin and can be made available for use by your body. When it reaches its target, a small portion of your testosterone is converted into a more potent metabolite called dihydrotestosterone (DHT). Having some DHT is essential, but too much can cause male pattern baldness and prostate enlargement.

In healthy men, testosterone production drops approximately 1% to 3% a year after age 30. In addition, the production of SHBG increases, so the amount of free testosterone drops substantially (figure 3). In the last 20 years scientists have been starting to recognize this decline as more than just "getting old." Names for this condition have varied. Initially called "male menopause" or "andropause," more recently terms like Symptomatic Late-Onset Hypogonadism (SLOH) and Androgen Deficiency in the Aging Male (ADAM) have been used. Behind all these confusing names and acronyms is the growing realization that declining levels of testosterone and other hormones are not "normal." Unlike menopause in women, however, men do not experience abrupt hormonal declines but a more subtle, gradual and variable decline.

Figure 3

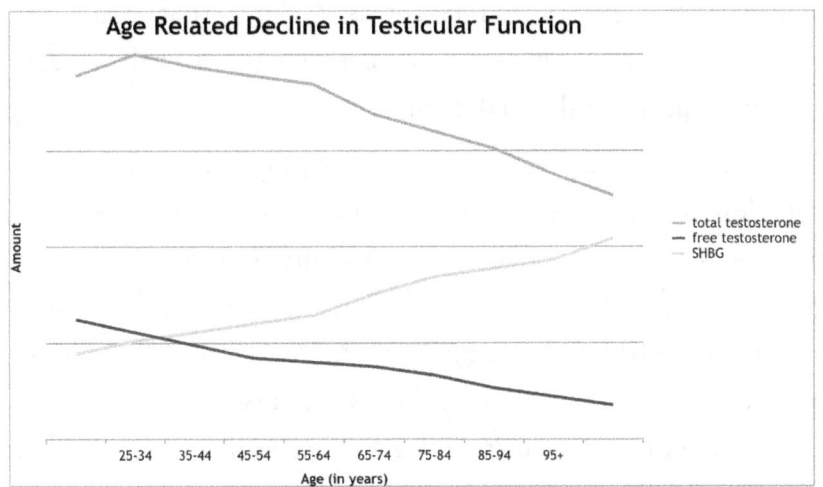

Like other endocrine deficiencies, declining testosterone causes changes in a man's metabolism with short and long-term effects. Although most people think of testosterone only affecting the genitals, the changes caused by declining testosterone levels affect every organ system. These changes include a decrease in bone density, decreased sexual desire, softer erections, decreased number of morning erections, increases in mood and psychological disorders, increased visceral (belly) fat, decreased muscle mass, an increase of diseases like cardiovascular disease and an increased risk of premature death.

Testosterone deficiency has a large number of effects on the brain. The brain is capable of producing its own testosterone and receptors for testosterone abound throughout the brain. These receptors appear to affect not merely sexual longing but also cognitive function. We are just beginning to understand the effects on the brain when free testosterone is reduced.

Elderly men in one study that had higher levels of bioavailable testosterone did better on three tests that are designed to find brain damage or dementia. Another type of impact is on specific kinds of thinking tasks. Declining testosterone reduces the type of thinking called "spatial cognition." This consists of tasks that require attention to objects in three-dimensional space like visual perception, object perception, and visual memory.

Sexual desire and interest is, not surprisingly impacted by testosterone levels. In fact, decreased libido with no other cause is a standard symptom that is looked for in deciding if a man has clinically significant decreased testosterone. Men with decreased testosterone also have more trouble getting or maintaining a good quality erection. Several small studies have shown that testosterone supplementation in older men results in both increases in libido and in a higher sense of well-being and satisfaction.

Testosterone also appears to both help protect and heal nerve cells in the brain. In laboratory studies, testosterone protects neurons from attack by a variety of possible toxins. It also helps heal severed nerves and produces other chemicals that help nerves re-grow after injury.

The general effects of testosterone are well known. It helps build muscle, bone, and other tissue. When these effects wane, mobility, strength, endurance, co-ordination, and other aspects of physical capability wane. The loss of independence, depression, obesity, and overall frailness we associate with old age are partly a consequence of this decline of the anabolic effects of testosterone.

Wanting to stay strong isn't merely vanity or machismo, it is a predictor of how aging will affect overall health. Men of all ages that have higher testosterone levels have better physical capacity as measured by physical fitness tests. Other effects on health outcomes are just as important. Men given testosterone supplementation have reduced body fat, increased lean muscle mass, and increased grip strength. They also gain upper and lower body strength and aerobic endurance. They have lower rates of bone loss and higher bone mineral density, so their bones are stronger.

The changes in the amount of body fat are important for two reasons: not only does testosterone reduce overall fat, but it specifically reduces "visceral" fat. The medical term is Visceral Adipose Tissue (VAT) but visceral fat is also called abdominal fat or organ fat. It is the fat that is located inside the abdomen instead of just under the skin where most fat deposits are located. Packed in among and around the abdominal organs, visceral fat is associated with a much greater risk of cardiovascular disease, diabetes, hypertension, cancer and atherosclerosis.

The common link in these changes appears to be suppression of a substance called adiponectin. Adiponectin is produced by fat cells in visceral fat stores, but adiponectin production generally goes down as the amount of visceral fat increases. As adiponectin production goes down, the risk of type 2 diabetes, obesity, atherosclerosis, fatty liver disease, and metabolic syndrome increases.

Testosterone supplementation increases both overall lean body mass and reduces visceral fat in older men.

Visceral fat's link to diabetes is also mediated through the same adiponectin. By increasing the effectiveness on insulin, higher adiponectin blood levels lower the risk of diabetes. Not surprisingly, men with lower testosterone levels have higher diabetes risks.

One thing that has been a surprise to many in the medical community is the way testosterone appears to lower cardiovascular risk. Because women before menopause have a lower risk of heart disease, it has been thought that estrogen provides some protection to the cardiovascular system. It was also assumed that this meant that testosterone was somehow antagonistic to the cardiovascular system.

This assumption was seemingly supported by the increased risk of heart attacks and strokes even in very young men abusing anabolic steroids. Together, these factors caused a great deal of resistance to the idea of supplementing waning testosterone levels.

By contrast, when men with lowered amounts of testosterone are studied, the risk of heart disease is increased over normal men, not decreased. Men that have coronary artery disease have lower levels of testosterone than men without blocked arteries. No study so far, in fact, shows a relation between higher testosterone and coronary artery disease. Neither do increased testosterone levels from supplementation lead to increased heart disease. This over-turns years of dogma and leads to the question of can testosterone supplementation help men with cardiovascular disease? In several leading medical centers, including Cedars Sinai in California, testosterone supplementation is being used with good results in men with heart failure.

Fortunately, men with decreased testosterone and coronary artery disease do show improvement when given testosterone supplementa-tion. Angina frequency and intensity are reduced, they tolerate exer-cise longer before experiencing chest pain, and have improved mood. Biochemical risk factors such as lipid profiles and insulin levels also show improvement.

To speak of mood and testosterone naturally returns to the subject of sexual function. As I said earlier, testosterone supplementation can increase sexual desire, but what about sexual capability? In normal men, during an erection more testosterone is available to the penis while overall testosterone in the blood also increases slightly. In men with erectile dysfunction, testosterone doesn't show the same response.

Erectile dysfunction can have many different causes: circulation problems, medications, psychological issues, and more. In psychological cases, testosterone tends to be in the normal range, while it is reduced in other cases. In men with erectile dysfunction and low testosterone levels, supplementation improves sexual function in a number of ways. It increases the number and quality of erections, and treated men also report more and better intercourse and increased sexual satisfaction.

Testosterone therefore alleviates or reduces many of the negative consequences associated with aging. Despite the multitude of significant health benefits and the volumes of studies refuting old assumptions, as I touched on in the last chapter, testosterone therapy remains controversial for many doctors due to fears about prostate cancer and heart disease risks.

Prostate cancer is the second most common cancer in men worldwide. One common treatment option is called androgen deprivation therapy (ADT), which aims to deprive prostate tumors of testosterone and similar hormones. This has a proven ability to shrink prostate tumors, leading to a suspicion that high testosterone or testosterone supplementation could create new prostate tumors.

On the contrary, there so far is no evidence that the levels of testosterone differ significantly between men that go on to develop prostate cancer and men that don't. This finding has been shown in over 18 different studies enrolling more than 8,000 men, all showing that testosterone levels have no clear relationship to developing prostate cancer. A more recent study showed that cancer mortality actually decreased as testosterone levels rose, with the men having the highest levels having the lowest number of cancer deaths.

Although not yet routine, there is a growing list of specialists that are treating selected men with testosterone following successful treatment of prostate cancer in order to restore their quality of life. In the limited number of cases thus far, none of the treated men have suffered a recurrence of their cancer. And men with low risk prostate cancer, with or without treatment, may be suitable candidates for testosterone therapy. This is certainly something that would need to be discussed on an individual basis.

Testosterone supplementation can both extend life and improve the quality of life in aging men. There are men that shouldn't be given testosterone such as men with aggressive prostate cancer, active liver disease or history of serious blood clots, but many other men can benefit greatly. The biggest obstacle to more widespread use of testosterone has so far been conservatism and misinformation. For men that are experiencing aging symptoms, however, I feel these should not be barriers to appropriate hormonal therapy.

Human Growth Hormone

Human Growth Hormone (HGH) may be the most controversial medication a doctor can prescribe in the United States today. HGH is responsible for rejuvenating and repairing all tissues in your body. As your HGH declines, it orchestrates many of the changes of aging. Changes like loss of muscle tone, wrinkles, energy decline and excess fat gain.

But add HGH back, and you reverse some of these unpleasant consequences of aging.

Starting about 20 years ago, research began suggesting that HGH declines as we age and that it has a large number of positive health effects beyond merely controlling skeletal growth, as it was shown it could fight aging symptoms if given as a supplement to adults.

Unfortunately, unlike almost all other drugs approved for use by the FDA, doctors are not allowed to prescribe HGH for the many conditions for which they feel it is appropriate. This makes HGH even more stringently controlled than many potentially addictive medications.

One of the reasons for controversy is that, like anabolic steroids, HGH has been abused by athletes as a performance-enhancing drug. Given this controversy, I should start by discussing what HGH does in the body and why it is so important for maintaining health in aging.

Human growth hormone is released by the anterior pituitary gland and when it reaches other tissues causes the production of chemicals called "insulin-like growth factors" (IGF). IGF's promote cellular growth, promotes injury healing to the muscles and bones, and causes more dietary and body fat to be used as energy for the body.

Like testosterone, HGH levels drop as we age. Every decade HGH production drops approximately 11%. As HGH levels drop, calories from the diet are burned less efficiently and deposited in the body. Diminished secretion of HGH reduces lean muscle mass, increases fat deposition, and thins the skin.

When people who have decreased HGH production due to aging are given daily HGH treatment, muscle mass goes up and body fat goes down. Even better, these changes are sustained for 5 years with minimal side effects. Other effects include an increase in bone density and bone strength, a decrease in both total cholesterol and LDL cholesterol (often called "bad cholesterol").

Excessive body weight and body fat are linked to most of the common causes of death once we get past middle age. Reducing excess fat and weight are therefore important concerns for maintaining overall health and living longer and better. Obese men and women given low-dose HGH lost weight, and analysis showed all the lost weight was from fat. Considering that HGH helps metabolize fat stores, this is not surprising, but it is significant.

As with testosterone, HGH aids in losing VAT --- the fat packed in among and around the abdominal organs. Reducing this fat has almost a synergistic effect. That is, losing one pound of visceral fat improves overall health and lifespan more than losing one pound of subcutaneous fat.

Another reflection of the improvement HGH gives fat metabolism is the change in what is called a "lipid profile." In people treated with HGH, total cholesterol, triglycerides, and LDL cholesterol are all reduced, and HDL cholesterol is increased. These changes are all positive and directly indicate the body is metabolizing fat in a healthy way.

HGH achieves all these changes in fat metabolism multiple ways. In fat cells, HGH stimulates breaking down stored fat and releasing it into the blood stream. In muscles, HGH causes these released fats to be taken up more efficiently and turned into fuel. In the liver, HGH enhances absorption of the triglycerides so they aren't used to make lipoprotein molecules.

All these changes in fat metabolism are interesting, but mean little if they don't have actual, measurable effects on your life. Fortunately, there is a way to measure directly the risk of cardiovascular disease. Atherosclerosis is the hardening of the arteries caused by deposition of cholesterol and other materials in the artery walls. Left unchecked, these plaques can cause complete blockage of an artery, leading to a stroke or heart attack.

There is a test that directly measures the progress of atherosclerosis by using ultrasound to determine the thickness of the walls of the carotid arteries called the carotid intima-media thickness test (CIMT). People that have low production of HGH have worse lipid profiles and also have thicker carotid artery walls. It suggests that supplementing HGH for a person with low production will reduce or possible even reverse the progression of cardiovascular disease.

These changes are enhanced further when HGH is combined with sex hormones (testosterone in men, estrogen and progesterone in women). When taken together in this manner, the strength, body composition, and weight improvements were even more pronounced than HGH alone.

The other part of total body mass that HGH affects is, of course, bone. Growth hormone is important for gaining height in children and teenagers, but that does not mean it is irrelevant to adults. When HGH production declines, bone replacement activity slows down and the density of the bones also declines. This makes the larger bones weaker and more susceptible to fracture.

Bones are constantly undergoing a rebuilding process called turn-over. In a healthy person, turnover is balanced between the cells that build new bone (called osteoblasts) and the cells that break down old bone (called osteoclasts). In children or healing bone, osteoblasts are more active and bones grow. In osteoporosis and related diseases, osteoclasts are more active and bones become thinner and more brittle. HGH stimulates the osteoblasts and suppresses the osteo-clasts, causing strengthening.

When these people are given HGH supplements, their bone density increases. They not only stop bone loss, but add new strength to their bones. The improvement is almost immediate and sustained for long periods.

What all this comes down to is this: HGH declines as we age, HGH decline causes (at least partly) many of the stereotypical effects of aging, HGH supplementation in people that have low production of the hormone improves or reverses these changes.

Although it remains controversial, used judiciously, HGH supplementation can remodel the aging body. Aside from HGH injections, there are several injectable peptides that stimulate your body to produce and secrete more of its own HGH. Tessamorelin is the most effective of these peptides. Many physicians, including myself, believe this is a more natural solution. The use of these peptides are also not restricted as much as HGH itself. Whichever way you increase HGH levels, it helps people's bodies become stronger, lighter, and healthier.

Estrogen

Why am I talking about estrogen, of all things, in a book on improving male performance? The truth is, estrogen has a large number of health effects in men, some good and some bad. Normally, men have 20% -33% less estrogen than woman before menopause. That doesn't mean estrogen is not a necessary part of a healthy endocrine balance in men.

In women, of course, estrogen is produced in the ovaries and is the primary hormone responsible for the development of secondary sexual characteristics during puberty and is responsible for regulating fertility as an adult. Because men lack ovaries, and testosterone is the primary regulator of male development and fertility, men usually assume they have no estrogen.

Men also produce estrogen, mostly in fatty tissue. Fat cells have an enzyme called aromatase that converts testosterone into estrogen. There are two different forms of estrogen in men; estradiol and estrone, with estradiol being more predominant.

What does estrogen do in men, though? To start with, there are estrogen receptors in the testicles and estrogen is necessary for proper development of the male reproductive tract in puberty and for maintaining fertility in adulthood. Estrogen is also very important for controlling bone growth and bone health in men, and may play a role in cardiac health in older men. There are also estrogen (and progesterone) receptors in the brain, where it helps protect against brain injury, neurodegeneration, and mental decline.

Unlike testosterone, estrogen levels do not automatically drop as men age. Older men, in fact, often have higher levels of estrogen than younger men both because of increased efficiency of the conversion of testosterone into estrogen and because of increases in the amount of fatty tissue.

In addition to producing estrogen, fatty tissue also has estrogen receptors. If these receptors are not functioning properly, then the amount of fatty tissue increases. This, in turn, causes even higher production of estrogen and a lower uptake in the local tissues, releasing more estrogen to the bloodstream where it can affect other parts of the body.

Another source of estrogen in men is environmental. Without realizing it, you are exposed every day to environmental chemicals that mimic estrogen, called "xenoestrogens." The term literally means "foreign" estrogens and refers to estrogen-like compounds that are not produced by your body.

Some xenoestrogens are similar to regular estrogen and some are very different, but they all have the ability to stimulate or interfere with the same receptor pathways as regular estrogen. Industrial chemicals like some insecticides, detergents, water repellents, and solvents are potent disruptors of estrogen. Other chemicals that affect estrogen metabolism are industrial contaminants like PCB's and bisphenol-A (the chemical that was recently banned from plastics in children's products).

A surprising source of exposure to xenoestrogens is through environmental exposure to hormones. The volume of oral contraceptives consumed by women in this country, and other Western countries, is enormous. A portion of the estrogen in these contraceptives, or their metabolic products, is discharged into wastewater every day. From there, they can make their way into the environment through the wastewater treatment processes.

Synthetic xenoestrogens, while significant in modern society, are actually dwarfed in importance by estrogen-mimicking chemicals from other sources. Estrogen-like plant chemicals called phytoestrogens are present in many foods. The foods that contain the highest levels of phytoestrogens are nuts and seeds, soy products, cereals, legumes, and meat products.

Excess estrogen can cause a number of difficulties, particularly in older men. Estrogen can interfere with testosterone receptors, reducing the ability of testosterone to stimulate arousal and sensation and also causing a loss of libido. High levels can also interfere with the production of sperm, reducing fertility.

Excess estrogen has been linked to increased risk of prostate cancer.

Estrogen also has a role in the linkage of obesity to diabetes. For multiple reasons, obesity increases the risk of diabetes, but one of the ways that this risk is increased is through the activity of aromatase.

As I mentioned before, excess body fat increases the amount of aromatase available to convert testosterone to estrogen. Men with lower levels of testosterone have a greater risk of developing Type 2 diabetes.

Estrogen is also linked to bone health in men. During puberty, the level of estrogen in both men and women helps determine when the growth plates of bones fuse, stopping the growth of the bones. In elderly men, the higher the level of estrogen, the healthier their bones are. Men with higher estrogen have denser bones and their bones have more turnover. The higher rate of turnover indicates that the cells that remove old bone and lay down new bone are more active and overall healthier. This is also important because these cells are what help heal fractures.

High estrogen levels can also wreak havoc on your mood, memory, mental clarity, and energy. For most of my male patients, I want a ratio of 10 to 20 parts testosterone per one part estradiol in blood levels.

There are steps you can take to reverse the damage from environmental exposures that include, washing your vegetables and fruits before you eat them, trim visible fat from meat before cooking (the chemicals and hormones from the feed collect in the fat), avoid processed meats, (because they have fat ground in), eat hormone-free food and free range animals whenever possible, avoid sugars and processed carbohydrates like bread, cereals, and pasta (they make your body release excess insulin, which builds fat and stimulates feminizing estrogen), eat more cruciferous vegetables like broccoli, cauliflower, Brussel sprouts, and cabbage (these help you excrete excess estrogen).

To rid your body of excess estrogen, you can take estrogen-regulating supplements such as indole-3-carbinol (I3C) or diindolylmethane or DIM.

By taking advantage of the hormones we already produce, we can miraculously turn back the clock on the aging process. And the best part is that this can happen without the use of synthetic drugs. In a way, the miracle is that we now understand how to apply these human hormones intelligently.

Chapter 5
Optimize Your Nutrition

Year after year, many people resolve to lose weight. But every year, the majority of people making weight loss resolutions fail to achieve them.

The result of these failures is highlighted in a study by the Centers for Disease Control that estimated the body fat percentage of a typical American woman to be 40% and the typical American man at 28% based on a six-year analysis of data.

Although body fat percentages vary somewhat by age, the optimal body fat for women is 18-22% and for men 15-18%.

Whatever the excuse for why a weight loss program fails, the core reason is that the person attempting to lose weight did not change their lifestyle as it related to their nutritional habits.

Attempting a temporary diet is a sure path to failure, because the dieter is not committing to changing the negative actions that caused the unwanted weight gain.

Another problem with diets is that they aim for weight loss, not fat loss. Too many of these diets are nutritionally unbalanced. The body needs each class of nutrients in the right proportions: fats, carbohydrates, and proteins, in addition to vitamins, and minerals. The typical American diet lacks sufficient protein and contains excessive amounts of highly processed carbohydrates and unhealthy fats.

"Crash diets," the kind promoted in magazines with titles like "Lose 10 pounds by next week!" are even worse. Most of the weight lost in these diets is water. All body tissues are mostly water, so water weight loss is part of all diets. By removing almost only water weight, however, you are not changing any of the risk factors associated with excess body fat.

Worse yet, most crash diets call for essentially starving yourself. This sends signals to the body that you are going through a period of famine. The body responds by increasing your fat stores when normal eating is resumed, to prepare for the next "famine." The end result, then, is exactly the opposite of what is intended. Instead of becoming healthier and lighter, you add weight and frustration.

In fact, men that have gone through multiple periods of weight loss and weight gain (referred to as weight cycling), store more fat in their abdomen. Abdominal (or visceral) fat is a risk factor for many negative health consequences including cardiovascular disease, diabetes and premature death. Having a higher amount of abdominal fat is directly linked to higher levels of "bad" cholesterol (LDL) and lower levels of "good" cholesterol (HDL). It is also linked to insulin resistance, and metabolic syndrome.

Genomic testing is available to help personalize recommendations for you. While our understanding of the technology is not quite at a point where every detail of your intake can be analyzed with respect to your DNA blueprint, many of the critical metabolic processes that can alter the way your genes are expressed can be modified with the right dietary and nutraceutical interventions.

In addition to dieting and hormone balance, an appropriate exercise regimen needs to be a part of your high performance lifestyle makeover.

We are able to accurately measure and quantify the accumulation of visceral adipose tissue (VAT) using the latest CoreScan™ technology during Total Body Composition analysis on our Lunar Prodigy DEXA scanner.

Chapter 6
Exercise Smarter

Starting an exercise program is a necessary part of a healthy lifestyle change. Granted, this is no major revelation. Burning more calories than you eat seems like a fairly obvious recipe for weight loss, but the body is more complex than that. The question then becomes: How should you exercise for maximal fat loss and optimal long-term changes in body composition?

Many magazine articles, trainers, coaches, and even the recommended heart charts on exercise equipment all suggest that you should exercise at a moderate intensity for long durations. Conventional wisdom has said that this is the best intensity for two reasons: 1.) Because you burn more fat at this intensity and; 2.) Because it avoids the dreaded lactic acid buildup. This conventional prescription, however, is based on outdated ideas about how the body responds to exercise.

Your body can utilize several different fuel sources; carbohydrates, fat and proteins, and varies the proportion of each depending on the intensity and duration of an activity. For the first couple of minutes of exercise, your body uses energy stored in muscles as something called ATP – the most readily available source of energy. But your supplies of stored ATP are limited and must quickly be replenished from other fuels. After 2 to 3 minutes, your body switches to carbohydrates stored in muscle tissue as glycogen. This lasts for 15 to 20 minutes before you start to incorporate fat as a fuel source to generate ATP.

Claims that moderately intense exercise burns more fat are based on studies that showed increased consumption of calories from fat over long workout periods. The idea was to favor "long and slow" exercise, like a marathoner, instead of "short and fast" exercise, like a sprinter.

Research in recent years, however, is showing that the assumptions behind this recommendation are not entirely correct. To the extent that a person exercising in this range is burning a greater proportion, the effect is small. But burning fat during exercise is not the way to achieve long-term changes in body composition and become leaner.

Moderate intensity durational exercise just doesn't stress the energy-supplying systems efficiently. The body has two paths to turn stored energy into work: the aerobic and anaerobic systems. The aerobic system uses oxygen to break sugars, fats and protein into energy. Anaerobic system works when not enough oxygen is reaching muscle cells. You can get a very high-energy output from this system but not for very long. When you are using your anaerobic system, you are building up reserve capacity in your heart, expanding your lung volume, triggering the production of growth hormone and melting away fat. Moderate-intensity aerobic training improves aerobic power without changing anaerobic capacity, but high-intensity training improves both anaerobic and aerobic systems significantly.

Other drawbacks with this durational exercise method are numerous. On a psychological level, this type of moderate exercise is monotonous. This is important because boredom is one reason that people often give for quitting exercise programs. If the workout is boring, is it any wonder most people consider going to the gym an unpleasant chore?

Higher intensity effort is more challenging and achieves exercise goals in less time. More intense efforts also require more concentration, creating more interest in the workout.

The most important limitation is that, like crash dieting, "long and slow" exercise can have a counter-productive effect. Drawing preferentially from fat stores tells your body you need that fat. The body replenishes these "necessary" fuel stores the next time you eat, and becomes more efficient at both using and maintaining fat. Top-level endurance athletes expend enough total calories to overcome this handicap, but most of us find ourselves fighting an uphill battle.

Interestingly, while they may not accumulate fat, it has been noted that the muscles of marathon runners actually shrink. When the muscle biopsies of marathon runners were analyzed, researchers found their muscle fiber size had decreased and atrophied. One has only to look at elite marathon runners to see the paucity of their muscle mass, which can accelerate some negative effects of aging.

We see patients actually gain weight in many long duration, moderate-intensity exercise programs. Short bursts of exercise tell your body that storing energy as fat is inefficient, since you never exercise long enough to utilize the fat during each session.

Carbohydrates, which are stored in muscle rather than fat, burn energy at high rates. Exercising for short periods will use these carbohydrates and burn much more fat after exercising while you replenish the carbohydrate stores. Short interval exercise maximizes fat "after burn." High-intensity exercise stresses both the aerobic and anaerobic systems. By doing so, it forces the body to recover and rebuild once the effort ends. In fact, studies show that high-intensity short duration exercise increases fat oxidation long after the exercise is completed. The most important effects of exercise occur after, not during, your exercise session. If done correctly, it can affect your metabolism for several days afterward.

Prolonged endurance exercise causes inflammation and generates free radicals, which cause damage to cells and possibly accelerate aging. Excess free radicals are especially damaging because they directly attack DNA, which can cause mutations, cell death, or cancer.

Free radicals also cause other unwanted reactions leading to cell damage, such as breaking down cell walls, interfering in protein synthesis, and more. In such ways free radical damage, also called "oxidative stress" is involved in diseases like atherosclerosis and liver disease.

Free radicals produced by "long and slow" exercise, such as a marathon, can also damage "good" cholesterol (HDL) for up to 4 days after the exercise is over, further increasing heart disease risk. It is not uncommon for a marathon runner to collapse and die suddenly at an endurance event.

Other unwanted effects of prolonged moderate intensity exercise include things like destruction of bone mass. Male long-distance runners have lower bone mass and higher bone turnover than control groups, which indicates bone loss. Another study of male long-distance runners showed that they had lower levels of testosterone and higher levels of the stress hormone cortisol, and that these levels did not return to normal after a break in training.

With all these dire effects, it may be easy to conclude that exercise can do almost as much harm as good. That isn't the case at all, of course. The right exercise for the right person is still an effective part of the lifestyle changes that will improve your overall health.

What each person making such changes needs is an exercise program that treats them as an individual. Books, health magazine articles, etc. give recommendations based on what works for large groups, but what if you do not conform to the "average" person?

The pros and cons of different interventions, and combinations of interventions, should be weighed and balanced. What you need, in essence, is an exercise prescription.

Depending on your individual goals, genomic testing can guide you toward the ideal combination of exercise intensity and duration to improve your results. Fortunately, there are professionals that can help cut through this morass of information. Once a plan is in place, committing to long-term changes is a key attitudinal adjustment. By focusing on making changes to the way you treat food and exercise instead of "going on a diet" you are much more likely to be successful.

Chapter 7
Make Recovery a Priority

Exercise training is the stimulus for gains in aerobic capacity, endurance, strength, muscle mass and power to take place. But doing that hard work alone does not guarantee the results you want. Your improvements really occur outside of your workouts, during your recovery. If you do not recover well, you won't see the results you expect.

All activity that we undertake and all bodily functions use energy (in the form of ATP). A byproduct of that energy usage is the generation of free radicals that can cause oxidative stress. Very generally, endurance exercise produces a far greater number of free radicals (up to 100x more) than shorter duration exercise. Intense cognitive work for several hours can use a comparable amount of energy to running a marathon.

At any given time, you have a finite amount of ATP your body can produce. If your exercise consumes a disproportionate amount, that would not leave enough for other bodily processes to function properly. Similarly, if you push yourself physically or mentally without sufficient recovery, your performance will drop and your results will tank. That is, if you don't rest or sleep enough, you will not be able to regenerate sufficiently. The repair and recovery process also requires energy (ATP) and if it is not available it cannot happen.

Contrary to much of what you may have been lead to believe, free radicals are not always harmful. Without free radicals you cannot make energy. Antioxidants are good but you can have too much of them. If you fully suppressed all free radical production, you would die. Some free radicals are essential in the body for inflammation (healing), immune function and repair.

Avoiding the activities that produce oxidative stress is not practical or desirable, so the question is how can we assist the body to repair the damage and recover so that performance can remain high?

It is a delicate balance. The younger, fitter and healthier you are, the greater capacity you have for repair. Even at its best, you cannot repair all of the damage, hence the aging process. So the harder you train the more dedicated you need to be to clean eating, taking supplemental antioxidants and allowing yourself sufficient rest to recover. There is exciting new technology on the horizon, which promises to augment the natural biological signal to regenerate and repair oxidative stress damage and ultimately boost cellular activity. If it lives up to its promise, it should help you recover faster and more effectively so you can derive greater benefit from your workouts.

Chapter 8
Are You Losing Muscle Mass?

"Normal" aging is typically accompanied by easier weight gain and, along with declining hormones and decreased physical activity can reduce muscle mass, lead to frailty and a higher prevalence of metabolic disorders. This insidious, age-related loss of muscle mass is called sarcopenia.

In many respects, sarcopenia is to muscle what osteoporosis is to bone. The typical American gains one pound of fat and loses a half-pound of muscle yearly between age 30 and 60. Deterioration of muscle and loss of muscular strength is a major reason the elderly lose mobility and cannot remain living independently.

Although muscle mass and strength both decline with age, the declines do not correlate directly. Muscular strength can be maintained for a decade or more after a noticeable amount of muscle mass has been lost.

The most accurate predictor of functional decline in later life is a measure of muscular work, such as "power;" or the amount of work a muscle can accomplish in a given amount of time. Strength is the maximal force a muscle can generate. Power implies a component of velocity. For example, muscular strength may help reduce injuries from falls in the elderly but if one trips, it is the immediate rapid movements that can prevent the fall.

Well-recognized risk factors for sarcopenia include increasing age, diminishing hormones, low levels of physical activity, and inadequate nutrition. Recent studies implicate oxidative stress as a significant risk factor for muscle wasting.

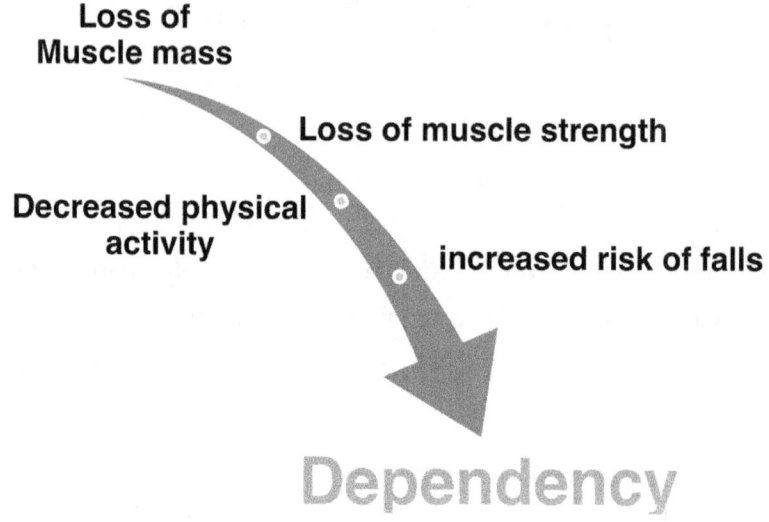

Mitochondria, the microscopic power plants within every cell, convert fuel into energy. One consequence of this energy production is the formation of free radicals, or reactive oxygen species, which are potentially harmful if produced in excess.

Mitochondrial efficiency also plays a role in free radical defense. Exercise is the most proven method of increasing the efficiency of existing mitochondria as well as stimulating the production of additional mitochondria. It can also be stimulated by nutritional interventions.

Resveratrol, a compound found in red wine, has been associated with anti-cancer activity, protects the heart, has antioxidant and anti-inflammatory activity. Resveratrol activates a class of genes called sirtuins that improve the efficiency of metabolism, reduce cellular stress and are associated with longevity. L-arginine alpha ketoglutarate (AKG) promotes nitric oxide(NO) production. Nitric oxide is produced by a layer of cells lining blood vessel walls and regulates the flow of blood to tissues. When released, it causes the blood vessels to relax and expand, increasing blood flow and oxygen to tissues. NO is necessary for a man to achieve an erection and is the pathway affected by medications like Viagra. NO has recently been found to directly regulate the oxygen supply to mitochondria. Alpha Lipoic Acid (ALA) increases energy expenditures, improves insulin sensitivity, and reduces appetite. It functions by activating an enzyme (AMPK), the "fuel sensor" enzyme for the body, and is the pathway through which ALA increases mitochondrial production.

Increased mitochondrial density and number allow more energy to be produced, and more muscular work to be performed.

Lack of muscle mass or mitochondrial density predisposes individuals to weight gain, insulin resistance, type-2 diabetes, metabolic syndrome and frailty.

Research reveals that resistance training can counteract the decline in skeletal muscle mass, maintain motor skills and reduce the risk of metabolic syndrome. Mitochondria within skeletal muscle are the primary target for carbohydrate and fat metabolism to produce energy.

Maintaining adequate muscle mass and mitochondrial density is a proactive measure to offset the risk factors related to metabolic syndrome, such as obesity, elevated blood pressure and hemoglobin A1C levels (a measure of blood glucose control over time). It has been widely known that resistance training is critical in preventing osteoporosis. It is now clear that resistance training should also be recommended for type-2 diabetes and metabolic disorders.

Rapid weight lifting, or an interval-style resistance program, has been shown to increase muscular power output more dramatically than traditional resistance training. It is a misconception that higher intensity exercise is riskier and only suited to younger individuals. An intensive exercise training program improves measures of physical function, such as strength, gait, balance and oxygen uptake better than a low intensity home exercise program in older adults.

Generally oxygen uptake declines 10-15% per decade after age 20; with an accumulation of body fat and a decrease in habitual physical activity accounting for about half of that age-related decrease. Oxygen uptake is a measure of aerobic fitness. Deterioration in aerobic fitness may result in a loss of independence in later life by limiting one's physical endurance.

A recent study demonstrated that long term regular exercise was associated with improved preservation of telomere length, which, as you will see in the next chapter, determines aging at a cellular level. Proper mitochondrial function is also crucial for aerobic performance. As the site of energy production in the cell, mitochondria are critical for the function and endurance properties of muscle.

So what's the message here? Exercise is a key determinant of how well you will age, your risk for developing chronic diseases, how well and how long you will live and how long you can remain independent as you age. But, it is not enough to do just one type of exercise, nor is it enough to occasionally go for a stroll. Exercise requires you to put in some work, sweat, and get out of breath. Just remember to allow enough time to recover adequately between exercise sessions.

Maintaining muscle mass, muscular strength, muscular power and endurance are all essential to maximizing performance and aging more youthfully.

Chapter 9
Age Reversal Is Possible

Pick up any health related magazine and you are sure to find some "anti aging" article. To be sure, there is no shortage of dubious promises and untested remedies to increase longevity that are peddled to the naïve or ill-informed. But recent scientific discoveries are unraveling the secrets of aging on a cellular level and may identify ways to slow it down. The obvious benefit to that is the longer we can maintain our youth, the less functional decline we will encounter and the less likely we will develop a chronic disease and die. The mechanism by which aging can be controlled lies in our understanding of cellular aging. At the end of each strand of DNA in our body is a protective endcap called a telomere. They represent your cellular biological clock and are the strongest indicator of how quickly you age. Telomeres protect the vital information in our DNA.

When we are born, telomeres are at their greatest length. As we age, our cells divide, resulting in the telomeres becoming progressively shorter. Eventually the telomeres become too short to perform their job, resulting in the death of the cell.

In addition to naturally shortening with age, telomeres have been shown to shorten in response to stress and poor lifestyle choices such as smoking, obesity, lack of exercise and an unhealthy diet. There is also a growing body of scientific evidence showing the association of age-related diseases, such as heart disease, cancer, and dementia, and shorter telomeres. At any age, shorter telomeres dramatically increase your risk of serious disease and premature death. You will look and feel older.

Telomere length can be measured with a simple blood test. Several labs perform telomere testing, but there is only one lab in the world, Life Length Labs, that can provide you with a measure of critically short telomeres. From a clinical perspective, that is the most significant parameter and the reason we use Life Length Labs at Alternity Healthcare.

To optimize human performance, knowing your telomere length becomes crucial. Remember, improving your overall performance is dependent upon the performance of your cells. By optimally maintaining the health of your cells, you create an environment that conducive to cellular repair, maintenance of telomeres and results in a longer health span. The rate at which your telomeres shorten is directly related to your lifestyle (nutrition, exercise, stress, and sleep), and with better lifestyle choices telomere shortening may be slowed. Recent studies have suggested that an "age-reversal" effect is possible. That is, even if your telomeres are short, there are things you can do to boost their length, make your cells act younger, avoid age-related problems and restore your youthful vigor… at any age!

Nutrients with a positive effect on telomere biology include high dose, high quality omega-3 fatty acids (EPA & DHA), vitamin A, gamma tocotrienols (a form of vitamin E), and vitamin D3 with K2. A unique, patented supplement, TA-65, has been shown in a 2016 study to lengthen telomeres by activating an otherwise dormant enzyme, telomerase, that repairs and restores telomeres.

Here is an example of a patient in our peak health program whose telomeres lengthened with a customized, targeted nutraceutical regimen including TA65, and appropriate lifestyle modifications. This "age reversal" corresponded to a substantial improvement in health, vitality and happiness.

	Range	7/6/2015	7/6/2016	7/3/2017
Median Telomere Length	Kb	9.2	9.5	10.4
Average Telomere Length	Kb	10.9	11.1	12.2
Critically Short Telomere Length	Kb	4.4	4.9	5.5
percentile rank		25th	40th	75th
Estimated biological age	years	78	77	72
Chronological age	years	74	75	76

There is compelling evidence that whatever your age, having longer telomeres is associated with better health and vitality. It is a number that everyone should know about themselves. This is something that I urge all of my patients to have done.

Your DNA Blueprint

Certain guidelines generally apply to a healthy lifestyle—eat lots of fresh vegetables, fruits and natural foods, reduce the intake of sugar and processed foods, and drink plenty of water. But any one-size-fits-all dietary program will inevitably fall short of providing the optimal nutritional needs unique to your personal genetic makeup.

Your DNA creates the blueprint for all the functions in your body. Passed down from our parents, each person has 46 chromosomes (23 pairs): one pair from your mother, and one from your father. Your unique combination of chromosomes creates your DNA that contains genetic variations called polymorphisms.

Identifying and evaluating small genetic variations called SNPs, or single nucleotide polymorphisms, can provide more individualized information than ever before. By knowing you from the inside out, personalized health strategies can be created that are specifically tailored to your unique genetic and biochemical needs.

Epigenetics refers to the interactions of your DNA with lifestyle factors, such as diet and physical activity, and environmental factors that can activate or suppress gene expression. It is not changing your DNA, it is the understanding of what genetic hand you have been dealt and developing personalized interventions that help optimize performance in every aspect of your life.

Using this intimate level of information allows us to truly personalize our assessment of your sleep, hormones, detoxification, nutrition, nutraceutical supplementation, weight loss, athletic performance

Care and Feeding of Your Brain

You are frantically looking for your keys or your phone but can't remember where you put them down. Memory lapses can be frustrating and seem to occur with increased frequency as you get older. You may blame it on your busy life or work demands, but secretly may wonder if you are losing some of your faculties. Has this happened to you?

Medical advances have dramatically increased the likelihood of surviving into the period of life that has been associated both with wisdom and mental decline. Especially if you have taken good care of your physical body, it is becoming more and more common to enter into the eighth and ninth decades of life in generally good physical health. An unforeseen consequence may very well increase the probability that your body will outlive your mind.

Recent experiments in neuroplasticity—the ability of the brain to change in response to experience—reveal that the brain is capable of altering its structure and function, and even generating new neurons well into old age. Think of your brain as a dynamic, adaptable system. The neurons respond to environmental factors and stimulation. By stimulating your mind, you preserve your memory, and can even restore the clarity you had in your youth. As stated in earlier chapters, hormone balance, and specifically testosterone plays a vital role in maintaining brain health.

Maintaining cognitive competency is crucial for personal independence and quality of life. Factor in the growing evidence that how one lives in earlier stages of life, including our food choices, affects cognitive aging; we all should be paying a little more attention to what we feed our brains.

It is now clear that significant cognitive decline is not an inevitable consequence of advanced age. Several recent studies have demonstrated an association between eating a Mediterranean-style diet and slower cognitive decline in the elderly. A well-designed prospective study published in the American Journal of Nutrition analyzed data from a continuing study of 3,790 Chicago residents 65 and older that began in 1993. The researchers tested the subjects' mental acuity at three-year intervals, and tracked their degree of adherence to the Mediterranean diet on a 55-point scale. High scores for adherence to the diet were associated with slower rates of cognitive decline, even after controlling for smoking, education, obesity, and hypertension.

Another study, presented at the American Academy of Neurology's April 2010 meeting in Toronto, analyzed the diets of 712 New Yorkers. MRI brain scans taken an average of 6 years later revealed brain infarcts in one third of the study participants. Brain infarcts are small areas of dead brain tissue caused by silent strokes that may show no symptoms. Recent research has suggested that brain infarcts may be responsible for decreasing cognitive function as we age. In this study, the group who most closely followed a Mediterranean-style diet was 36% less likely to have the damaging brain infarcts than the group who least followed the diet, and moderate followers were 21% less likely to have damage than the lowest-tier group. A third study published in the February 2009 issue of Archives of Neurology found that eating a Mediterranean diet was possibly associated with a reduced risk of developing mild cognitive impairment (MCI) and of MCI advancing to Alzheimer's disease.

Benefits of the Mediterranean diet may be due to the it's positive impact on cholesterol levels, blood sugar levels, vascular health, or inflammation reduction; all of which have been linked with cognitive impairment.

Relaxation is just as vital for maintaining memory and cognitive abilities. If you are stressed or overworked all of the time, you are damaging your brain cells. Stress is a leading cause of mental deterioration because of the negative effects of excess cortisol (the stress hormone). Furthermore, as I stated in an earlier chapter on Recovery, intense mental activity can use the same amount of energy as running a marathon. Just as your body would breakdown from that level of activity if not given sufficient time for rest, repair and rejuvenation, your brain is no exception. Remember, there is a finite amount of energy that you can produce, of which some is required for repair. If there is not enough to do it all, your body and brain suffer. This really becomes important for you if you are that CEO, type-A guy trying to grow revenue for your company, run an ultra-marathon or Iron-man competition, all the while jetting around the world trying to survive on 4 hours of sleep. When you dance to the music…the piper must be paid!

Although there is a lot of data suggesting beneficial effects of a Mediterranean diet on a number of chronic medical conditions, diet alone is not the only factor. Diet is but one component of a healthy lifestyle that includes regular exercise, prevention or treatment of diabetes, hypertension, high cholesterol, obesity—if they exist, balancing hormones, avoidance of smoking and incorporating stress reduction strategies like regular massage, learning mindfulness or meditation techniques and taking vacations. All of these together give you your best chance to remain cognitively intact as you age.

Chapter 10
The High Performance Prescription

Welcome to the future of medicine. As an international concierge health company we work with men from around the world; some completely virtual, some remote and some locally in our Connecticut office. Whether you are one of our patients, clients or health participants, you will benefit from my extensive medical knowledge, expertise, coaching and guidance in a manner that suits your preferences and geographic practicality.

The Process

Creating a truly personalized experience and powerfully sustainable health transformation for you requires a high degree of customization and attention to detail for each person. As such, we can only work with a limited number of motivated individuals at a time.

If you want to be proactive about your health, are open-minded, coachable and success-oriented, and, most importantly, are ready to accelerate your performance in every aspect of your life, I invite you to apply directly to work with me. The brief application can be found at: AlternityHealthcare.com/consult-application/

If you have questions you'd like to ask to help you determine if Alternity Healthcare is right for you, our patient coordinator is standing by to accept your call 860-561-2294 or you can schedule a free discovery consultation by clicking this link to the practice calendar AlternityHealthcare.com/become-a-patient/

High Performance Blueprint

In order to provide you with a personalized roadmap allowing you to access your highest level of performance, experience youthful vitality and optimized health, we utilize a unique 3-step process:

Step 1- DISCOVERY. To set out on the proper course, you must first know where you currently stand. We begin with an in-depth baseline evaluation to discover the unrecognized and underlying issues that may be interfering with performance and increasing health risks by taking into account your physiology, genetics, nutrition, sleep, stress, hormones, environment and individual goals. By using advanced lab diagnostics, including telomere analysis, gut micro-biome testing, selected genomic profiles, environmental toxicology, immunology, and oxidative stress markers, among others; it provides us a broader view of where you are as a human being.

Step 2 – TRANSFORMATION. With the information from your baseline evaluation, we use proven strategies to create a high performance roadmap enabling you to recapture the energy and vitality of your youth through individualized, precision lifestyle modifications that may favorably alter epigenetic expression so you can perform at your absolute best and magnify your impact.

Step 3 – TRANSCEND LIMITATIONS. With ongoing monitoring, feedback, coaching and support we empower you to expand your vision beyond self-limiting beliefs and transform your potential into exceptional performance in every aspect of your life. We are committed to helping you integrate sustainable solutions to increase energy, productivity and happiness, while reversing disease risks and issues that can impair your performance.

VIP Executive Assessment

If you have chosen one of our in-office VIP Executive Assessments, the "discovery" process will include the diagnostic data generated during your evaluation day. Going well beyond an "annual physical", you'll spend four to six hours of your day with us. This extensive evaluation focuses not only on the early detection of disease, but can identify physiologic dysfunction that could be impacting your performance and potentially lead to future disease.

Your VIP Executive Assessment will include special testing to measure lung function, arterial elasticity, central blood pressure, body composition and bone density. You will meet with a registered dietitian or nutritionist to analyze your eating patterns and supplement use, and an exercise physiologist to assess your fitness, flexibility, strength, movement patterns and determine your aerobic capacity through a cardiopulmonary exercise test. You will also complete a psychological screening and computerized cognitive assessment. A gourmet healthy lunch will be provided and you'll have extensive one-on-one time with me.

Results Analysis

There are many benefits that can be derived from the identification and management of the underlying factors putting your health at risk and impairing your peak performance potential. You'll improve resiliency, melt away body fat and regain muscle mass, experience firmer erections and heightened sexual pleasure, boost your memory and brain power, have better relationships with loved ones and experience lifelong vitality. Although different from individual to individual, you will typically begin to see the results of implementing your program recommendations within three to six months. As long as you remain committed to continue to follow our recommendations, your results should be sustainable for life.

No matter how healthy you think you are, there may be unrecognized, underlying risk factors detectable years before they become diseases when they may be more amenable to treatment. Furthermore, unless you are complacent with merely good enough, there are always things that could be improved in your quest to live your life as the best version of yourself.

Chapter 11
Real Results, Real People

Case Study 1

A 56-year old male presented with loss of libido and difficulty achieving a satisfactory erection. At the time of his assessment, he felt generally sad and grumpy, had diminished strength, reported low energy levels, and felt less healthy than 5 years prior. At that time he was taking 2 medications for blood pressure, 2 cholesterol/lipid medications, an antidepressant and sleeping pill. Our recommendations were as follows:

Exercise Prescription

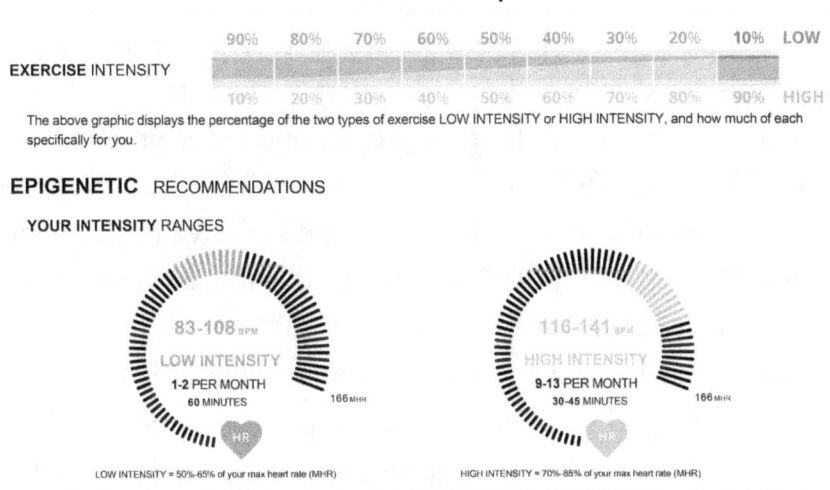

| 90% | 80% | 70% | 60% | 50% | 40% | 30% | 20% | 10% | LOW |

EXERCISE INTENSITY

| 10% | 20% | 30% | 40% | 50% | 60% | 70% | 80% | 90% | HIGH |

The above graphic displays the percentage of the two types of exercise LOW INTENSITY or HIGH INTENSITY, and how much of each specifically for you.

EPIGENETIC RECOMMENDATIONS

YOUR INTENSITY RANGES

83-108 BPM
LOW INTENSITY
1-2 PER MONTH
60 MINUTES
166 MHR

116-141 BPM
HIGH INTENSITY
9-13 PER MONTH
30-45 MINUTES
166 MHR

LOW INTENSITY = 50%-65% of your max heart rate (MHR)   HIGH INTENSITY = 70%-85% of your max heart rate (MHR)

In the illustrations above you will find your target heart rate for both LOW INTENSITY and HIGH INTENSITY exercise, the duration at which these exercises are performed and optimal weekly frequency.

Diet

CARB SENSITIVITY	LOW	MEDIUM	HIGH
	20% Males 20% Females	69% Males 66% Females	11% Males 14% Females

Reduce white flours and sugars and increase vegetables and fruits.

FAT SENSITIVITY	LOW	MEDIUM	HIGH
	36% Males 30% Females	22% Males 24% Females	42% Males 46% Females

Typically your body has challenges with weight loss, due to your homozygous proline variant. However, they can be overcome by your genotype's preferred program.

EPIGENETIC RECOMMENDATIONS

MACRONUTRIENT PROPORTIONS

25% FAT	40% PROTEIN	35% CARBOHYDRATE

Supplement Recommendations

FOUNDATION

CoQ10 CoQ10 is a compound involved in the body's production of adenosine triphosphate (ATP) which is an energy source for cells in the body and aids in functions like muscle contraction and protein production. *talk to your doctor before taking CoQ10 to be sure it does not interfere with any medications you are taking.

OPTIMAL HEALTH

Adrenal Support Excess exercise can cause health problems, especially if the diet is lacking in proper nutrition. Overtraining can signal the body to start burning muscle for fuel and store more fat, resulting in some weight gain. High intensity exercise is most effective when adrenal support is also taken into consideration.

Polyphenols Polyphenols are bioavailable flavonoids that play a role in preventative care. Polyphenols can interact at the cellular level by working in conjunction with fatty acids to keep the fats correct oxidative state. Polyphenols were generally viewed as antioxidants until the 90s, but have been shown to do much more than improve the state of oxidative stress. Polyphenols are found naturally, but the average diet is lacking. Resveratrol is a polyphenol nutrient known to activate signals that help break down your stored fat to use as fuel as well as boost your energy. Grapeseed extract is also a potent antioxidant and polyphenol.

By diligently following our prescribed program to improve his health, his mood improved, erectile function was restored and he was able to eliminate all medications except one blood pressure medication. Two years after starting his program, his life insurance agent noticed how much healthier he looked and suggested he get rerated, as his policy carried a $19,000+ premium due to his poor health. It was rerated at $2900 saving him nearly $16,000 on his life insurance premium. That does not take into account the savings on the medications he no longer had to buy and most importantly it does not factor in the "cost" of poor health or some catastrophic health crisis he is now less likely to experience. What is the true value of the peace of mind and improved quality of life?

In his own words…

When I came in to see Dr. Ebanks, he was blatantly honest about the changes I needed to make to get healthier. I realized that getting healthy was an important investment in the long-term success of my business. I have had great results. I have lost weight and feel much better than I have in the past. I eat much healthier, exercise regularly and sleep better than I have in years. There is one other interesting side benefit of getting healthier. Three years ago I needed to purchase a large amount of life insurance.. I was high risk. And to purchase $500,000 of additional insurance, it cost me a little over $19,000 annually. About 18 month after starting on my program, I visited with my insurance agent who met me at my office, came in and said: "you look great". We started talking about this one insurance policy that I have with a huge premium. He said, "why don't we put some feelers out to see if we could get you a better rate". Dr. Ebanks put a document of my current health data together, sent it in and we got a policy with a much more favorable outcome. I actually bought $650,000 of life insurance for $2900 per year. The savings was over $16,000 annually and a benefit I had never expected. So besides feeling better personally, my wallet feels a lot better also.

Case Study 2

A 40-year old male presented with complaints of fatigue, trouble recovering from a work out, and that those workouts were not as effective as in the past. He indicated that he no longer felt "young anymore." Using an analysis of his genomic data, we identified areas in his diet and exercise routine that were impairing his performance.

Exercise Prescription

EXERCISE INTENSITY

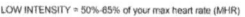

60%   70%   75%   65%   50%   **40%**   30%   20%   10%   LOW

10%   20%   30%   40%   50   **60%**   70%   80%   90%   HIGH

The above graphic displays the percentage of the two types of exercise LOW INTENSITY or HIGH INTENSITY, and how much of each specifically for you.

EPIGENETIC RECOMMENDATIONS

YOUR INTENSITY RANGES

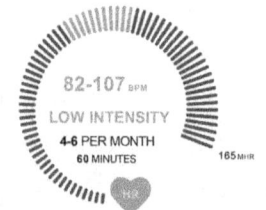

82-107 BPM
LOW INTENSITY
4-6 PER MONTH
60 MINUTES
165 MHR

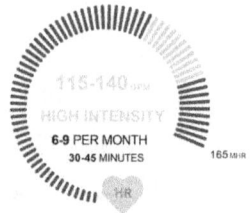

115-140 BPM
HIGH INTENSITY
6-9 PER MONTH
30-45 MINUTES
165 MHR

LOW INTENSITY = 50%-65% of your max heart rate (MHR)   HIGH INTENSITY = 70%-85% of your max heart rate (MHR)

In the illustrations above you will find your target heart rate for both LOW INTENSITY and HIGH INTENSITY exercise, the duration at which these exercises are performed and optimal weekly frequency.

Diet

CARB SENSITIVITY

LOW	MEDIUM	HIGH
20% Males	69% Males	11% Males
20% Females	66% Females	14% Females

Reduce white flours and sugars for weight loss. Maintain adequate glucose for sustained energy.

FAT SENSITIVITY

LOW	MEDIUM	HIGH
36% Males	22% Males	42% Males
30% Females	24% Females	46% Females

Typically your body has challenges with weight loss, due to your homozygous proline variant. However, they can be overcome by your genotype's preferred program.

EPIGENETIC RECOMMENDATIONS

MACRONUTRIENT PROPORTIONS

25% FAT	45% PROTEIN	30% CARBOHYDRATE

Supplement Recommendations

FOUNDATION

Crave Control Carbohydrate cravings have been directly associated with serotonin levels. Serotonin-releasing brain neurons are unique in that the amount of neurotransmitter they release is normally controlled by carbohydrate consumption--acting via insulin secretion. Studies show that carbohydrate cravers eat 800 or more calories a day than other people. Balancing serotonin levels can help reduce cravings.

Polyphenols Polyphenols are bioavailable flavonoids that play a role in preventative care. Polyphenols can interact at the cellular level by working in conjunction with fatty acids to keep the fats correct oxidative state. Polyphenols were generally viewed as antioxidants until the 90s, but have been shown to do much more than improve the state of oxidative stress. Polyphenols are found naturally, but the average diet is lacking. Resveratrol is a polyphenol nutrient known to activate signals that help break down your stored fat to use as fuel as well as boost your energy. Grapeseed extract is also a potent antioxidant and polyphenol.

OPTIMAL HEALTH

Omegas A blend of omega-3 and omega-6 fatty acids may be necessary due to the decrease of fats from your diet. Essential fatty acids (EFAs) aid in human metabolism and are necessary for proper function of the body's systems, including the skeletal and cardiovascular systems, with added benefits to brain function. They are not produced by the body so we must get EFAs from our diet.

Vitamin B complex Vitamin B12, folic acid and magnesium help support methylation. B vitamins also keep the nervous system in tune, enhance energy and aid in stress-relief. They are great for the eyes, skin and hair.

WEIGHT LOSS

BCAAs Leucine, isoleucine and valine provide nutritional support for individuals seeking optimal lean muscle mass. BCAAs will "trick" your body into thinking it has been replenished in proteins and begins using free fatty acids for energy, post workout. "Avoid consuming anything with carbohydrates for 90 minutes, post exercise (liquid or solid foods) as it will immediately stop fats being used for energy" (Take BCAAs if your initial goal is to lose weight.)

Providing him with personalized recommendations and coaching around stress management and sleep hygiene, allowed him to make the right modifications to optimize his results.

In his own words...

I never had a physician that looked at total prevention. My energy and libido were down but other doctors told me there was nothing wrong. I was impressed with Dr. Ebanks' approach. I felt like I could communicate with him and there was a level of mutual respect and understanding. He gave me an appreciation that there is another way to look at health and there are pretty simple means to improve health to make your life better. Finding out what my body's specific individual needs were has helped me get my life together. I feel like I did five years ago again. I have more energy, I can get more done, and I just feel better.

Case Study 3

A 60-year old entrepreneur presented with feelings that he was "past his prime." He was considering the sale of his business and retiring because he had lost the stamina and motivation to function at a high level. His diet was poor due to frequent eating out for business and he rarely exercised. Based on genomic data we tailored an eating program and exercise routine to improve his overall physical and metabolic profile.

Exercise Prescription

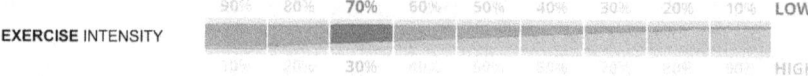

EXERCISE INTENSITY

90%	80%	**70%**	60%	50%	40%	30%	20%	10%	**LOW**

| 10% | 20% | 30% | | | | | | | **HIGH** |

The above graphic displays the percentage of the two types of exercise LOW INTENSITY or HIGH INTENSITY, and how much of each specifically for you.

EPIGENETIC RECOMMENDATIONS

YOUR INTENSITY RANGES

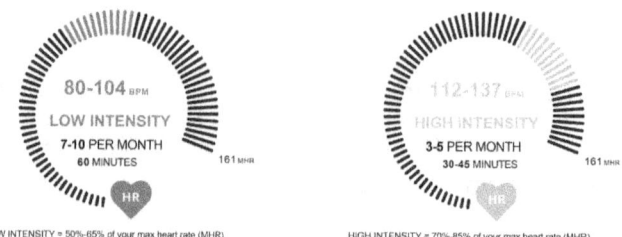

80-104 BPM
LOW INTENSITY
7-10 PER MONTH
60 MINUTES
161 MHR

112-137 BPM
HIGH INTENSITY
3-5 PER MONTH
30-45 MINUTES
161 MHR

LOW INTENSITY = 50%-65% of your max heart rate (MHR) HIGH INTENSITY = 70%-85% of your max heart rate (MHR)

In the illustrations above you will find your target heart rate for both LOW INTENSITY and HIGH INTENSITY exercise, the duration at which these exercises are performed and optimal weekly frequency.

Diet

CARB SENSITIVITY

LOW	MEDIUM	HIGH
20% Males	69% Males	11% Males
20% Females	66% Females	14% Females

Reduce white flours and sugars and increase vegetables and fruits.

FAT SENSITIVITY

LOW	MEDIUM	HIGH
36% Males	22% Males	42% Males
30% Females	24% Females	46% Females

Typically your body has challenges with weight loss, due to your homozygous proline variant. However, they can be overcome by your genotype's preferred program.

EPIGENETIC RECOMMENDATIONS

MACRONUTRIENT PROPORTIONS

20% FAT	**45%** PROTEIN	**35%** CARBOHYDRATE

Supplement Recommendations

FOUNDATION

Crave Control Carbohydrate cravings have been directly associated with serotonin levels. Serotonin-releasing brain neurons are unique in that the amount of neurotransmitter they release is normally controlled by carbohydrate consumption--acting via insulin secretion. Studies show that carbohydrate cravers eat 800 or more calories a day than other people. Balancing serotonin levels can help reduce cravings.

OPTIMAL HEALTH

Omegas A blend of omega-3 and omega-6 fatty acids may be necessary due to the decrease of fats from your diet. Essential fatty acids (EFAs) aid in human metabolism and are necessary for proper function of the body's systems, including the skeletal and cardiovascular systems, with added benefits to brain function. They are not produced by the body so we must get EFAs from our diet.

Polyphenols Polyphenols are bioavailable flavonoids that play a role in preventative care. Polyphenols can interact at the cellular level by working in conjunction with fatty acids to keep the fats correct oxidative state. Polyphenols were generally viewed as antioxidants until the 90s, but have been shown to do much more than improve the state of oxidative stress. Polyphenols are found naturally, but the average diet is lacking. Resveratrol is a polyphenol nutrient known to activate signals that help break down your stored fat to use as fuel as well as boost your energy. Grapeseed extract is also a potent antioxidant and polyphenol.

Vitamin B complex Vitamin B12, folic acid and magnesium help support methylation. B vitamins also keep the nervous system in tune, enhance energy and aid in stress-relief. They are great for the eyes, skin and hair.

WEIGHT LOSS

BCAAs Leucine, isoleucine and valine provide nutritional support for individuals seeking optimal lean muscle mass. BCAAs will "trick" your body into thinking it has been replenished in proteins and begins using free fatty acids for energy, post workout. "Avoid consuming anything with carbohydrates for 90 minutes, post exercise (liquid or solid foods) as it will immediately stop fats being used for energy" (Take BCAAs if your initial goal is to lose weight.)

Cardio Support The amino acids L-Arginine and L -Carnitine have both shown to increase blood flow to the muscles, and also aid in weight loss. L-Arginine increases activity of a protein that controls energy balance. It decreases the expression of genes that favor production of fats and glucose and increases the breakdown of fats. L-Carnitine is essential for fat metabolism and energy production. Either of these amino acids will offer great support.

By following our program, the patient gained 15lbs of muscle and lost 19lbs of fat. After working with him and restoring his vitality, he opted to expand his business, grew the revenue and several years later was able to sell the more profitable business and "retire" more comfortably. After retiring, he remained energized with his program and is currently planning to start a new business venture.

In his own words…

I met Dr. Ebanks at a conference where he was a featured speaker on executive health. His presentation intrigued me. He talked about unusual services and diagnostics that catch problems early, giving patients time to change, so they can avoid chronic problems. I was especially intrigued by the concept of telomere testing and repair. The longer your telomeres the longer your life expectancy. I have great genes, but I know that bad habits can mess that up. I have wonderful grand kids and I want to stick around a while. I opted for the top of the line "Executive Health Assessment". Since then, I have changed my diet and upped my activity level… In six months I lost 22 pounds, I have a lot more energy, and I feel better about myself… I had a bit gut, which might be considered normal for a 60-year-old, but I look and feel better now. I knew I had to do it. I was a willing candidate, and its working great, which makes it easier. I've decided I want to lose another

20 pounds, and I'm on track to do that. Dr. Ebanks is always available, and that's a big positive for me. I check in with him a lot. Some of the services he offers are expensive, but it's been worth every penny. In fact, I would do it again if it cost twice as much.

Meet Dr. Desmond Ebanks

D r. Ebanks is Founder and Medical Director of Alternity Health-care, LLC. He is a board certified Internal Medicine specialist, with over three decades of clinical experience in Internal, Emergency and Occupational Medicine. Dr. Ebanks has pioneered an innovative concierge model of care focused on identifying key biomarkers and physiologic measurements in order to maximize performance as a means of managing the aging process and addressing the root causes of disease and dysfunction.

Dr. Ebanks was an Assistant Clinical Professor of Medicine at New York Medical College and an Adjunct Clinical Professor of Medicine at Cornell University School of Medicine before launching Alternity Healthcare.

Dr. Ebanks graduated from Temple University School of Medicine and completed his residency training in Internal Medicine at Harlem Hospital, a Columbia University affiliate, and SUNY-Downstate Medical Center in New York. He earned his undergraduate degrees in Biology and Psychology from Syracuse University.

Together with his wife Cynthia, daughter Neena and Spanish Waterdog Amelia, Dr. Ebanks lives in Avon, Connecticut. When he is not working, Dr. Ebanks can be found relaxing with his family and friends, playing golf, tennis or basketball, traveling and enjoying jazz.

For more information about Dr. Ebanks' work and to subscribe to his blog, visit:

AlternityHealthcare.com

Follow him on social media:

www.facebook.com/AlternityHealthcare
www.twitter.com/AlternityHealth
www.linkedin.com/in/AlternityHealthcare

References

Albert SG, Mooradian AD. Low-dose recombinant human growth hormone as adjuvant therapy to lifestyle modifications in the management of obesity. Journal of Clinical Endocrinology and Metabolism. 2004 Feb;89(2):695-701.

Amin S, Zhang Y, Sawin CT, et al. Association of hypogonadism and estradiol levels with bone mineral density in elderly men from the Framingham study. Ann Intern Med. 2000 Dec 19;133(12):951-63.

Andreoli TE, Carpenter CCJ, Bennett JC, Plum F, eds., Cecil Essentials of Medicine, fourth edition, W. B. Saunders Company, Philadelphia, 1997

Appleby P, Key TJ. Endogenous sex hormones and prostate cancer: a collaborative analysis of 18 prospective studies. Journal of the National Cancer Institute. 2008 Feb 6;100(3):170-83.

Aversa A, Isidori AM, Spera G, et al. Androgens improve cavernous vasodilation and response to sildenafil in patients with erectile dysfunction. Clinical Endocrinology. 2003 May;58(5):632-8.

Bain J. Testosterone and the aging male: To treat or not to treat? Maturitas. 2010 Feb 12. [Epub ahead of print]

Baker JR, Bemben MG, Anderson MA, Bemben DA. Effects of age on testosterone responses to resistance exercise and musculoskeletal variables in men. Journal Of Strength And Conditioning Research. 2006 Nov;20(4):874-81.

Bates KA, Harvey AR, Carruthers M, Martins RN. Androgens, andropause and neurodegeneration: exploring the link between steroidogenesis, androgens and Alzheimer's disease. Cellular and Molecular Life Science. 2005 Feb;62(3):281-92.

Baum NH, Crespi CA. Geriatrics. Testosterone replacement in elderly men. 2007 Sep;62(9):15-8.

Becker AJ, Uckert S, Stief CG, et al. Cavernous and systemic testosterone plasma levels during different penile conditions in healthy males and patients with erectile dysfunction. Urology. 2001 Sep;58(3):435-40.

Bex M, Bouillon R. Growth hormone and bone health. Hormone Research. 2003;60 Suppl 3:80-6.

Binder E, Schechtman B, Ehsani A, et al. "Effects of exercise training on frailty in community-dwelling older adults: results of a randomized, controlled trial". .J Am Geriatr Soc. 2002 Dec;50(12):2089-91.

Blackman MR, Sorkin JD, Münzer T, et al. Growth hormone and sex steroid administration in healthy aged women and men: a randomized controlled trial. Journal of the American Medical Association. 2002 Nov 13;288(18):2282-92.

Boon WC, Chow JD, Simpson ER The multiple roles of estrogens and the enzyme aromatase. Prog Brain Res. 2010;181:209-32.

Calvo JA, Daniels, TG, et al. "Muscle-specific expression of PPAR(gamma) coactivator1(alpha) improves exercise performance and peak oxygen uptake". J Appl Physio 2008; 104:1304-1312

Caminiti G, Volterrani M, Iellamo F, et al. Effect of long-acting testosterone treatment on functional exercise capacity, skeletal muscle performance, insulin resistance, and baroreflex sensitivity in elderly patients with chronic heart failure a double-blind, placebo-controlled, randomized study. Journal of the American College of Cardiology. 2009 Sep 1;54(10):919-27.

Carruba G. Estrogen and prostate cancer: an eclipsed truth in an androgen-dominated scenario. J Cell Biochem. 2007 Nov 1;102(4):899-911.

Carruba G. Estrogens and mechanisms of prostate cancer progression. Ann N Y Acad Sci. 2006 Nov;1089:201-17.

Coward RM Simham J, Carson CC. Prostate-specific antigen changes and prostate cancer in hypogonadal men treated with testosterone replacement therapy. BJU Int 2009 May; 103(9): 1179-83.

Dubal DB, Zhu H, Yu J et al. Estrogen receptor alpha, not beta, is a critical link in estradiol-mediated protection against brain injury. Proc Natl Acad Sci U S A. 2001 Feb 13;98(4):1952-7.

Eaton NE, Reeves GK, Appleby PN, Key TJ. Endogenous sex hormones and prostate cancer: a quantitative review of prospective studies. British Journal of Cancer. 1999 Jun;80(7):930-4.

Endogenous Hormones and Prostate Cancer Collaborative Group, Roddam AW, Allen NE, Appleby P, Key TJ. Endogenous sex hormones and prostate cancer: a collaborative analysis of 18 prospective studies. Journal of the National Cancer Institute. 2008 Feb 6;100(3):170-83.

English KM, Mandour O, Steeds RP, Diver MJ, Jones TH, Channer KS. Men with coronary artery disease have lower levels of androgens than men with normal coronary angiograms. European Heart Journal. 2000 Jun;21(11):890-4. PMID: 10806012

Faloon W, As we see it; Why estrogen balance is critical to aging men, Life Extension Magazine, 2010 May

Fielding, RA, Katula, J, Miller, ME, Abbott-Pillola, K, at al. "Activity Adherence and Physical Function in Older Adults with Functional Limitations." Medicine & Science in Sports & Exercise. 2007 (November); 39 (11): 1997-2004

Frisch H. Growth hormone and body composition in athletes. Journal of Endocrinological Investigation. 1999;22(5 Suppl):106-9.

Fuller SJ, Tan RS, Martins RN. Androgens in the etiology of Alzheimer's disease in aging men and possible therapeutic interventions. J Alzheimers Dis. 2007 Sep;12(2):129-42.

Funahashi T, Nakamura T, Shimomura I, et al. Role of adipocytokines on the pathogenesis of atherosclerosis in visceral obesity. Internal Medicine. 1999 Feb;38(2):202-6.

Gómez JM, Gómez N, Fiter J, Soler J. Effects of long-term treatment with GH in the bone mineral density of adults with hypopituitarism and GH deficiency and after discontinuation of GH replacement. Hormone and metabolic research. 2000 Feb;32(2):66-70.

Gooren LJ. Endocrine aspects of ageing in the male. Molecular and Cellular Endocrinology. 1998 Oct 25;145(1-2):153-9.

Götherström G, Bengtsson BA, Bosaeus I, et al. Ten-year GH replacement increases bone mineral density in hypopituitary patients with adult onset GH deficiency. European Journal of Endocrinology. 2007 Jan;156(1):55-64.

Götherström G, Elbornsson M, Stibrant-Sunnerhagen K, et al. Ten years of growth hormone (GH) replacement normalizes muscle strength in GH-deficient adults. Journal of Clinical Endocrinology and Metabolism. 2009 Mar;94(3):809-16.

Götherström G, Svensson J, Koranyi J, et al. A prospective study of 5 years of GH replacement therapy in GH-deficient adults: sustained effects on body composition, bone mass, and metabolic indices. Journal of Clinical Endocrinology and Metabolism. 2001 Oct;86(10):4657-65.

Gruenewald DA, Matsumoto AM. Testosterone supplementation therapy for older men: potential benefits and risks. Journal of the American Geriatric Society. 2003 Jan;51(1):101-15;

Harley CB, Liu W, Blasco MA, Vera E, Andrews WH, Briggs LA, Raffaele JM. A Natural product Telomerase Activator as Part of a Health Maintenance Program. Rejuvenation Research. 2011 February; 14(1): 45—56.

Heine PA, Taylor JA, Iwamoto GA, Increased adipose tissue in male and female estrogen receptor-alpha knockout mice. Proc Natl Acad Sci U S A. 2000 Nov 7;97(23):12729-34. Proc Natl Acad Sci U S A. 2000 Nov 7;97(23):12729-34.

Hess RA, Bunick D, Lee KH, et al. A role for oestrogens in the male reproductive system. Nature. 1997 Dec 4;390(6659):509-12.

Isidori AM, Giannetta E, Gianfrilli D, Greco EA, Bonifacio V, Aversa A, Isidori A, Fabbri A, Lenzi A. Effects of testosterone on sexual function in men: results of a meta-analysis. Clinical Endocrinology. 2005 Oct;63(4):381-94.

Jang Y, et al. "Increased superoxide in vivo accelerates age-associated muscle atrophy through mitochondrial dysfunction and neuromuscular junction degeneration" FASEB Journal, 2009

Jankowska EA, Filippatos G, Ponikowska B, et al. Reduction in circulating testosterone relates to exercise capacity in men with chronic heart failure. Journal Of Cardiac Failure. 2009 Jun;15(5):442-50.

Jankowska EA, Rozentryt P, Ponikowska B, et al. Circulating estradiol and mortality in men with systolic chronic heart failure. JAMA. 2009 May 13;301(18):1892-901.

Jaskelioff M., Muller F.L., Paik J.H., Thomas E., Jiang S., Adams A.C., Sahin E., Kost-Alimova M., Protopopov A., Cadiñanos J., Horner J.W., Maratos-Flier E., Depinho R.A. Telomerase reactivation reverses tissue degeneration in aged telomerase-deficient mice. Nature. 2011;469(7328):102-106.

Johansen T, Malmlöf K. Treatment of Obesity Using GH. Metabolic Syndrome And Related Disorders. 2006 Spring;4(1):57-69.

Jørgensen JO, Rubeck KZ, Nielsen TS, et al. Effects of GH in human muscle and fat. Pediatric Nephrology. 2010 Apr;25(4):705-9

Khaw, KT, Dowsett, M, Folkerd E, et al. Endogenous testosterone and mortality due to all causes, cardiovascular disease, and cancer in men: European Prospective Investigation into Cancer in Norfolk (EPIC-Norfolk) prospective patient study. Circulation. 2007 Dec 4;116(23):2694-701.

Landsberg L. Body fat distribution and cardiovascular risk. Archives of Internal Medicine. 2008; 168(15):1607-8

Lange KH, Isaksson F, Rasmussen MH, et al. GH administration and discontinuation in healthy elderly men: effects on body composition, GH-related serum markers, resting heart rate and resting oxygen uptake. Clinical Endocrinology. 2001 Jul;55(1):77-86.

Lester SJ, Eleid MF, Khandheria BK, Hurst RT. Carotid intima-media thickness and coronary artery calcium score as indications of subclinical atherosclerosis. Mayo Clinic Proceedings. 2009 March;84(3):229-233

Li s, Shin HY, Ding e, et. al. Adiponectin levels and risk of type 2 diabetes: a systematic review and meta-analysis. JAMA : the Journal of the American Medical Association. 2009; 302(2)179-188

Makimura H, Stanley T, Mun D, Chen C, Wei J, Connelly JM, Hemphill LC, Grinspoon SK. Reduced growth hormone secretion is associated with increased carotid intima-media thickness in obesity. Journal of Clinical Endocrinology and Metabolism. 2009 Dec;94(12):5131-8.

Malkin CJ, Channer KS, Jones TH. Testosterone and heart failure. Curr Opin Endocrinol Diabetes Obes. 2010 Jun;17(3):262-8

Malkin CJ, Pugh PJ, Morris PD, Asif S, Jones TH, Channer KS. Low serum testosterone and increased mortality in men with coronary heart disease. Heart. 2010 Nov;96(22):1821-5. Epub 2010 Oct 19.

Malkin CJ, Pugh PJ, Morris PD, Kerry KE, Jones RD, Jones TH, Channer KS. Testosterone replacement in hypogonadal men with angina improves ischaemic threshold and quality of life. Heart. 2004 Aug;90(8):871-6.

Matthews J, Gustafsson JA. Estrogen signaling: a subtle balance between ER alpha and ER beta. Mol Interv. 2003 Aug;3(5):281-92.

Møller N, Jørgensen JO. Effects of growth hormone on glucose, lipid, and protein metabolism in human subjects. Endocrine Reviews. 2009 Apr;30(2):152-77

Morales A, Heaton JPW, Carson CC. Andropause: A misnomer for a true clinical entity. Journal of Urology. 2000 Mar;163(3):705-12.

Morgentaler A. Testosterone and prostate cancer: an historical perspective on a modern myth. Eur Urol. 2006 Nov;50(5):935-9.

Murray RD, Wieringa G, Lawrance JA, et al. Partial Growth Hormone Deficiency is Associated With an Adverse Cardiovascular Risk Profile and Increased Carotid Intima-Medial Thickness. Clinical Endocrinology. 2009 Dec 18.

Nelson LR, Bulun SE. Estrogen production and action. J Am Acad Dermatol. 2001 Sep;45(3 Suppl):S116-24.

Nilsson R. Endocrine modulators in the food chain and environment. Toxicol Pathol. 2000 May-Jun;28(3):420-31.

Nilsson S, Mäkelä S, Treuter E, et al. Mechanisms of estrogen action. Physiol Rev. 2001 Oct;81(4):1535-65.

O'Donnell AB, Travison TG, Harris SS, Tenover JL, McKinlay JB. Testosterone, dehydroepiandrosterone, and physical performance in older men: results from the Massachusetts Male Aging Study. Journal of Clinical Endocrinology and Metabolism. 2006 Feb;91(2):425-31.

Oh JY, Barrett-Connor E, Wedick NM, Endogenous sex hormones and the development of type 2 diabetes in older men and women: the Rancho Bernardo study. Diabetes Care. 2002 Jan;25(1):55-60.

Racz L, Goel RK. Fate and removal of estrogens in municipal wastewater. J Environ Monit. 2010 Jan;12(1):58-70.

Rajapakse N, Silva E, Kortenkamp A. Combining xenoestrogens at levels below individual no-observed-effect concentrations dramatically enhances steroid hormone action. Environ Health Perspect. 2002 Sep;110(9):917-21.

Rennie MJ. Claims for the anabolic effects of growth hormone: a case of the emperor's new clothes? British Journal of Sports Medicine. 2003 Apr;37(2):100-5.

Roddam A, et al. Endogenous Sex Hormones and Prostate Cancer: A Collaborative Analysis of 18 Prospective Studies. JNCI J Natl Cancer Inst (2008) 100 (3): 170-183.

Rosen RC, Wu F, Behre H, et al. Quality of Life and Sexual Function Benefits Effects of Long-Term Testosterone Treatment: Longitudinal Results From the Registry of Hypogonadism in Men (RHYME). J Sex Med 2017;14:1104–1115.

Rudman D, Feller AG, Nagraj HS, et al. Effects of human growth hormone in men over 60 years old. New England Journal of Medicine. 1990 Jul 5;323(1):1-6.

Rudman D, Kutner MH, Rogers CM, et al. Impaired growth hormone secretion in the adult population: relation to age and adiposity. Journal of Clinical Investigation. 1981 May; 67(5): 1361–1369.

Sandival L, Singaravelu G, Harley CB, et al. A Netural Product Telomerase Activator Lenghtens Telomeres in Humans: A Randomized, Double-Blind, and Placebo Controlled Study. Rejuvenation Res. 2016 Dec;19(6):478-484. Epub 2016 Mar 30.

Sattler FR, Castaneda-Sceppa C, Binder EF, et al. Testosterone and growth hormone improve body composition and muscle performance in older men. Journal of Clinical Endocrinology and Metabolism. 2009 Jun;94(6):1991-2001.

Sheridan PJ. Androgen receptors in the brain: What are we measuring? Endocrine Reviews. 1983 Spring;4(2):171-8.

Simpson ER, Zhao Y, Agarwal VR, et al. Aromatase expression in health and disease. Recent Prog Horm Res. 1997;52:185-213; discussion 213-4.

Simpson ER. Genetic mutations resulting in estrogen insufficiency in the male. Mol Cell Endocrinol. 1998 Oct 25;145(1-2):55-9.

Simpson ER. Sources of estrogen and their importance. J Steroid Biochem Mol Biol. 2003 Sep;86(3-5):225-30.

Sohoni P, Sumpter JP. Several environmental oestrogens are also anti-androgens. J Endocrinol. 1998 Sep;158(3):327-39.

Stellato RK, Feldman HA, Hamdy O, Horton ES, McKinlay JB. Testosterone, sex hormone-binding globulin, and the development of type 2 diabetes in middle-aged men: prospective results from the Massachusetts Male Aging Study. Diabetes Care. 2000 Apr;23(4):490-4.

Sternbach H. Age-associated testosterone decline in men: Clinical issues for psychiatry. American Journal Of Psychiatry. 1998 Oct; 155(10):1310-8.

Strasser B, Siebert U, Schobersberger W. "Resistance training in the treatmen of metabolic syndrome". Sports Medicine, 40(5):397-415. May 2010

Tancredi A, Reginster JY, Schleich F, et al. Interest of the androgen deficiency in aging males (ADAM) questionnaire for the identification of hypogonadism in elderly community-dwelling male volunteers. European Journal of Endocrinology. 2004 Sep;151(3):355-60.

Tangney C, Kwasny M, et al. Adherence to a Mediterranean-type dietary pattern and cognitive decline in a community population. Am J Clin Nutr December 2010 ajcn.007369

Tauchmanova L, Di Somma C, Rusciano A, et al. The role for growth hormone in linking arthritis, osteoporosis, and body composition. Journal of Endocrinological Investigation. 2007;30(6 Suppl):35-41.

Taxel P, Kennedy DG, Fall PM, et al. The effect of aromatase inhibition on sex steroids, gonadotropins, and markers of bone turnover in older men. J Clin Endocrinol Metab. 2001 Jun;86(6):2869-74.

Tenover JL. Testosterone replacement therapy in older adult men. International Journal of Andrology. 1999 Oct;22(5):300-6.

Tenover JL. The androgen-deficient aging male: current treatment options. Reviews in Urology. 2003;5 Suppl 1:S22-8.

Thompson LU, Boucher BA, Liu Z, et. al. Phytoestrogen content of foods consumed in Canada, including isoflavones, lignans, and coumestan. Nutr Cancer. 2006;54(2):184-201.

Traish, A., et al., Long-Term Testosterone Therapy Improves Cardiometabolic Function and Reduces Risk of Cardiovascular Disease in Men with Hypogonadism: A Real-Life Observational Registry Study Setting Comparing Treated and Untreated (Control) Groups. Journal of Cardiovascular Pharmacology and Therapeutics, 2017: p. epub.

Traish AM, Guay A, Feeley R, et al. The dark side of testosterone deficiency: I. Metabolic syndrome and erectile dysfunction. J Androl 2009;30(1):10-22.

Tritos NA, Biller BM. Growth hormone and bone. Current Opinion in Endocrinology, Diabetes, And Obesity. 2009 Dec;16(6):415-22.

Vijayakumar A, Novosyadlyy R, Wu Y, et al. Biological effects of growth hormone on carbohydrate and lipid metabolism. Growth Hormone & IGF Research. 2009 Sep 30.

Weise M, De-Levi S, Barnes KM, et al. Effects of estrogen on growth plate senescence and epiphyseal fusion. Proc Natl Acad Sci U S A. 2001 Jun 5;98(12):6871-6.

Werner C, Furster T, et al. "Beneficial Effects of Long Term endurance Exercise with Leukocyte telomere Biology. Circulation. 2009;120:S492.

Wespes E, Schulman CC. Male andropause: myth, reality, and treatment. International Journal of Impotence Research. 2002 Feb;14 Suppl 1:S93-8.

White HK, Petrie CD, Landschulz W, et al.. Effects of an oral growth hormone secretagogue in older adults. Journal of Clinical Endocrinology and Metabolism. 2009 Apr;94(4):1198-206.

Wu FC, von Eckardstein A. Androgens and coronary artery disease. Endocrine Reviews. 2003 Apr;24(2):183-217.

Yaffe K, Lui LY, Zmuda J, Cauley J. Sex hormones and cognitive function in older men. Journal of the American Geriatric Society. 2002 Apr;50(4):707-12

Yarasheski KE. Growth hormone effects on metabolism, body composition, muscle mass, and strength. Exercise and Sports Science

Zitzmann, M. (2009) Testosterone deficiency, insulin resistance and the metabolic syndrome. Nat. Rev. Endocrinol. doi:10.1038/nrendo.2009.212